Zero Sugar Diet

Your Guide to a Sugar Free Diet With Recipes and Allergy Alternatives

Published by Digital Superheroes Publications

Book Description

Your stomach rumbles, and you think about grabbing a quick bite to eat. You glance up at the clock. It's 10:00 in the morning, and you think about how you have just eaten breakfast only a short while before. But then, lunch seems so far away.

How is it that you are hungry already? You think back to what you had for breakfast.

You were in a hurry this morning so you grabbed a scone and a latte from your favorite coffee shop on the way to work. But, that should have kept you satisfied, shouldn't it have?

Then again, you are usually hungry around this time, regardless of your breakfast – a doughnut, toast with jelly, your favorite cereal. You always drink your coffee to get you going in the morning. Cream and sugar is the best.

So, what's the problem?

If this sounds like a typical morning to you, sugar is very likely a culprit in your life. It is estimated that more than two-thirds of adults exceed their daily sugar recommendations by two or three times.

How do you cut this cycle? How do you break free from the sugar monster?

That's where this book comes in. In it, you are going to learn exactly what you need to do to cut the sugar out of your life, and enjoy the zero sugar diet. You will feel better, look better, sleep better, and live better. Guaranteed!

- **Learn how to start the zero sugar diet and stick with it**
- **Learn the benefits of the zero sugar diet and what it can do for you**
- **Get started with recipes that are sugar free and offer allergy alternatives**
- **And much, much more!**

Contents

Introduction

Sugar. It's everywhere. From the sugar in your coffee creamer to the sugar in the doughnut at the office to the sugar that is hiding in your favorite fruit drink, you have a sweet tooth that is being fed often, and well. It may surprise you how many forms sugar comes in.

You know that sugar can be bad for you. You've heard that it can cause tooth decay, it can cause weight gain, and it can cause diabetes. But, did you know that sugar can cause far more harmful things than even these?

That's right. Tooth decay can lead to cardiovascular problems. Sugar can lead to fatty liver problems and even obesity. Sugar can even be a direct cause of cancer in some people. Not only that, but sugar is largely responsible for your belly, your love handles, your blemished skin, and your premature aging.

The more you read on the list, the more you think about how bad sugar is for you, and how you should cut back – or completely cut it out of – your life.

Perhaps you know that you have a problem with sugar. Perhaps you are thinking of the soda you drink every day or every couple of days, the jelly you put on your toast, or the candy that you hide in the bottom of your drawer.

Or perhaps you don't think you have a problem with sugar at all. Perhaps you think that you are doing pretty well because you don't see the word sugar listed on the back of the foods you are eating. Perhaps you don't drink soda or eat candy.

Surprisingly, even if this does describe you, you may not be out of harm's way when it comes to sugar. Sugar comes in many different forms, and just because you don't see the word sugar on the back of the ingredient list, it doesn't mean that you aren't at risk.

Virtually any ingredient you see with the suffix -ose is a sugar, and it brings with it the harmful side effects that sugar causes. Regardless of how much sugar you think you are eating, you may be just as at risk as someone who knows they eat too much.

So what are you going to do? How do you kick this sugary habit and enjoy the healthy lifestyle you have been dreaming of?

You have come to the right place. In this book, you are going to discover the zero sugar diet, and learn how you can cut this harmful substance out of your life for good.

It doesn't matter if you have food allergies, if you have a raging sweet tooth, or if you merely don't know where to begin. I am going to put you on the right track to eliminating your sugar filled diet, and help you break the cycle of sugar in your own life.

If you are ready to dive into a healthy way of living, sleep better, experience fewer health problems, and live life for all that it's worth, you need to give up sugar – and I am here to show you how.

Let's get started.

Chapter 1 – Zero Sugar Diet: An Overview

Cakes, doughnuts, candies, desserts – needless to say, we all have a sweet tooth at least to some extent. From the glazed doughnuts for breakfast to the ice cream and cheesecake after dinner, who can say no to a sweet treat?

Perhaps if our only sugars came from these sweets we wouldn't have a problem, but the fact of the matter is that most people eat far more sugar and sweets than they ought to, and it's wreaking havoc on our health.

Obesity, diabetes, tooth decay, and a plethora of other health problems are considered normal, even among those who don't indulge in that extra slice of cake after dinner.

But why is this?

So many parents and so many people are incredibly careful about how much sugar their children eat. They aren't allowed to have soda, ice cream is limited, and they only purchase cereal that isn't sugar-coated.

While these are all healthy options, it they don't even begin to touch the issue. This is because sugar is a hidden culprit, and can be found in nearly everything – especially processed foods.

There are over 56 different kinds of sugars that are being added to everyday foods.

You will see these listed on the ingredient level as:

Sugar, sucrose, glucose, dextrose, rice syrup, carob syrup, corn syrup, barley malt, honey, fruit syrup, brown sugar, date sugar, blackstrap molasses, agave nectar, cane sugar, rice syrup, and many, many more.

Now, in a world that is becoming more concerned about sugar intake, you may have been told that some forms of sugar are better for you than others. While this may be true to an extent (and that is a very small extent,) you must realize that all sugars are going to cause your blood sugar levels to spike then drop again.

Another thing to take note of is that the earlier you see a sugar listed in the ingredient list, the more of that sugar is in the product you are reading about. For some foods, as you can imagine, have more sugar in them than anything else.

If sugar causes so many health problems, why do manufacturers insist on adding so many sugars to the foods they produce?

Even though there are some companies that are trying to cut back on the amount of sugar they place in their food, there are still many, many more that are continuously adding sugars to their products.

Is this a malicious act? Or is it something else?

To understand why these companies are adding sugar to their foods, you must understand what sugar does for food.

First of all, taste. Sugar adds a sweetness to foods that you may not even realize are sweetened. Pasta sauce, canned foods, yogurts, and even some meats' flavors are enhanced by the added sugars. Sugars also help add colors to certain foods, or enhance the colors of certain foods, making them more appealing to the consumer.

Sugar is also responsible for the density and textures of certain foods. It helps to ferment other foods, and it works as a preservative. If there is enough sugar added, the food will be more shelf stable and therefore last for a longer period of time than if the food didn't contain any sugar at all.

With this in mind, it's clear that manufacturers won't likely give up adding sugar to their foods any time soon.

Sugar and sugary derivatives are inexpensive and easy to add to foods, and compared to other kinds of preservatives, they are a somewhat healthier option. However, sugar consumption does come at a cost, and you must understand what putting that amount of sugar into your body is doing.

As I said, sugar is largely responsible for such things as obesity, tooth decay, and diabetes, but there are even more health risks associated with eating too much sugar.

An overload of sugar can be harmful to the liver, causing it to turn the sugars into fat on the body, but not just on the body, an overload of sugar can cause nearly the same effects on the liver as alcohol abuse.

The zero sugar diet is a diet that seeks to cut out as much added sugar as possible.

The American Heart Association recommends that you limit your sugar intake to no more than ninc tcaspoons per day if you are a man and six teaspoons per day if you are a woman.

Now, it is important to note that this is counting *added* sugars, not naturally occurring sugars. Fruits, vegetables, and many other natural foods have some sugars already in their makeup. These sugars are not what you have to watch out for, as your body automatically uses these sugars and converts them into useful energy.

The added sugars are the sugars that are not naturally occurring, and come in the forms of the other sugars that I have listed already.

We have already discussed why you should avoid these sugars, but in the next chapters I am going to show you the rich benefits that come from avoiding sugar, as well as give you recipes to get you started on your own sugar free diet.

Chapter 2 – Why Go Sugar Free? The Benefits of a Zero Sugar Diet

If you are considering going sugar free, you are not alone. Many people in society are trying to cut back on the sugar they are consuming, if not cut it out completely. As you have seen in the last chapter, there are many adverse side effects that come from eating too much sugar – many illnesses and chronic diseases can result.

However, cutting back or eliminating sugar from your diet because of the adverse side effects should not be the only reason you choose to remove this substance from your life. There are countless benefits that come from living the sugar free lifestyle.

That's right, not only can you expect to avoid a plethora of adverse side effects, but you can also expect to benefit in a variety of ways.

Perhaps the first and largest benefit you are going to experience from giving up sugar is weight loss.

As I have already pointed out, an excess intake of sugar overloads the liver, and not only leads to a fatty liver, but also leads to excessive fat being stored on the body. When you give up sugar, you aren't going to be overloading your body with too much of the substance any longer, meaning you will automatically lose weight, without having to put forth any extra effort.

Your skin will clear up, and appear to be more vibrant – almost instantly.

Many people who have given up sugar have reported that their skin clears. It doesn't matter if they are suffering from acne, dark spots, uneven skin tone, or what their blemish is, cutting back or eliminating the sugar in their diet has helped their skin clear up, and remain clear.

You will no longer obsess over food or battle food cravings throughout the day.

Studies have shown that sugar is as addictive as tobacco or nicotine – something that is a real wake up call to many people who consume sugar on a regular basis. This is why many people who consume a lot of sugar find themselves craving some sort of snack or treat shortly after consuming a meal.

This is especially true if you are used to adding sugar to your coffee in the morning, eating cereals that are sugar coated, or spreading that extra thick amount of jelly on your toast in the morning.

You will find that your aches and pains disappear.

People who quit sugar report that they no longer suffer from muscle or joint pain. Sugar has been directly associated with inflammation, and may give you the feeling that you have ants crawling around under your skin.

Cutting out the excess sugar in your diet will help your body eliminate this inflammation, and leave you feeling a lot better.

You will enjoy a stabilized mood and may even experience less anxiety, depression, and irritability.

Sugar intake has been associated with many mood disorders, even depression and anxiety. While giving up sugar may not cure your mood entirely, it will help with your mood swings and some of your anxiousness.

While it isn't entirely clear why sugar is linked to such moodiness, those who cut back on sugar do report that they feel a better sense of well-being than those who consume excess sugar.

You will sleep better at night.

The spikes in your blood sugar will inevitably give you more energy at the time, but it will throw off your sleep cycle during the night. If you find that you are having a difficult time sleeping at night, you should honesty take a look at your sugar intake – odds are you are eating it in excess.

You will have more energy throughout the day.

Remember what I said about sugar spiking your insulin levels? This phenomenon works as a cycle. First, your blood sugar goes up, which gives you a lot of energy and makes you feel like you can go for hours.

But then the crash hits. This is when your blood sugar levels drop below what they were before, making you feel sluggish and fatigued. As a result, many people find themselves reaching for another cup of coffee or a soda – something that they consider to be a pick-me-up (yes, the caffeine does help) but they are launching their insulin levels once again.

This vicious cycle keeps you constantly reaching for more and more sugar, keeping you enslaved in the same state you are in right now.

You will look younger and age better.

Remember what I said earlier about sugar affected the blemishes on your skin? Well it is also responsible for aging your skin – even prematurely. Cutting out sugar will not only cut back on the amount of money you are spending at the grocery store, but it's also going to cut back on the money you spend on cosmetics to stay younger.

All the while you are going to look younger and feel better – a complete win all around.

As you can see, there are far more benefits to quitting sugar than there are to consuming it. But, the concept of giving up sugar while nice in theory, can immediately feel overwhelming.

After all, when you flip over the product and see all the sugars listed on the back, it can be easy to feel like you no longer have any options as to what you can eat or drink. Don't worry. There are, in fact, dozens of options you have to choose from.

All it takes is a matter of changing your habits, and knowing which foods have less sugar, as well as which foods have no sugar at all. With time and practice you will catch on to what foods you can eat and which you should avoid, and it will all come as second nature.

Chapter 3 – How to Start a Zero Sugar Diet

The day you decide to start your zero sugar diet is an important one. It's the day you have decided to change your life. However, starting a zero sugar diet is easier said than done, and will require deliberate effort on your part.

The first step you must take in starting your zero sugar diet is to rid yourself of all the excess sugar in your home.

As I have said, sugar is addictive, and it isn't going to take long before you find yourself craving the sweetness. Just as you can't expect to give up alcohol if you have beer in the house, you can't expect to give up sugar if you have a sugar bowl or candy sitting on your counter.

Go through your kitchen and be ruthless. Clear out all the food you have that has added sugar, as well as the sugar itself. This includes the sauces, the pre-packaged foods, and all the inherently sweet things you have. Rid your cupboards of the candy, the desserts, and the ice creams, as well as the dessert mixes that you have yet to bake.

Read through all the ingredient lists you have on hand, and make a list of the foods you have that fit into your new diet plan. Though there are dozens of foods that have added sugars, you will be able to find alternatives if you look hard enough, and you may even have these alternatives in your pantry already.

The key to success on the zero sugar diet is to kick the sweet tooth you already have, and to form habits that will keep you with your diet in the future.

By understanding which foods you can have versus the foods that are filled with things you don't want to eat, you arm yourself with the knowledge you need to stick with this diet in the long term, and turn it into your new way of life.

When you decide to go zero sugar, you will lose weight, and you will experience the benefits you wish to experience.

However, as soon as you quit this diet, you are going to find yourself in the same boat as you were before. In order for you to enjoy the benefits of this diet in the long term is to not treat this as a diet, and instead to treat it as a new lifestyle.

Donate the food that you aren't keeping to the local food pantry or food share.

Going zero sugar is going to be one of the best things you can do for your health, but you must also understand that there is a lot of hunger and need, even locally. When you decide to go sugar free, help the other locals in your family by donating the food you aren't keeping, and help ease the burden on others. Perhaps they will also make the decision to cut out sugar down the road, but for now, you may be the blessing they have been looking for.

Take this food down to the pantry or donate it as soon as possible. The first few weeks of your sugar free diet is are going to be the hardest, and you don't want any temptation to be in the house.

But what about those who have food allergies? With a diet that is already restricted by food allergies, how are you going to cut out sugar?

It's overwhelming enough when you are trying to cut out sugar without any prior restrictions, but what about those who have food allergies on top of it? Nut allergies, dairy allergies, egg or fish allergies – you may have one or all of these. These make it harder for you to eat a well-balanced diet as it is, so it can be even more intimidating for someone who is going to also cut out sugar.

Intimidating? Yes. Difficult? Yes. Impossible? No.

In this modern world, there are a lot of choices for food alternatives, regardless of the dietary restrictions you have. Unfortunately, you do have to keep an eye on these foods, even if they do offer foods that are within your dietary preferences.

For example, you may be lactose intolerant and able to drink nut milks, but if you aren't careful with the nut milks you choose, you may easily be consuming 12 added grams of sugar in a single 8 ounce serving!

Many people who are allergic to eggs or milk will turn to protein bars that are dairy and egg free, only to find that these bars have more sugar in them than a can of soda. Even conventional pre-packaged "diet" foods are laden in sugar, largely due to the preservation powers sugar possesses.

So, while you may think that you are doing your body a service by avoiding the foods you are allergic to, you may not actually be doing as well as you could be.

Regardless of what you are able to eat on a day to day basis, going with the zero sugar diet is going to do your health wonders. For someone with more restrictions than others, the zero sugar diet may be a little more expensive to follow than how you are currently eating, but trust me, it is going to be worth it.

After all, your health is worth far more than you can put a price on, so don't be afraid to pursue a diet that is a little more difficult to follow than one that is easy but doesn't leave you feeling the way you want to feel.

And don't feel like you will be unable to enjoy the foods you eat. As I have said before, it's simply a matter of the habits you form that shape the outcome of what you are eating.

You will see by the recipes I have provided that you will have plenty of options when it comes to everyday foods, plus any alternatives you may have.

Whether you can eat anything you like or you have dozens of restrictions, sugar free is still the best option you can choose for your mind, body, and soul.

Chapter 4 – The First Week: What to Expect

Whenever you start anything new, or whenever you are quitting something (sugar is an addiction, after all!) you need to know what to expect. Many people who have tried to give up sugar experience adverse side effects – at first. And, without expecting these to happen, they don't realize they are natural and to be expected, therefore they give up.

With that in mind, I am going to prepare you for what you can expect in the initial stages of cutting out sugar. Some of it will feel great, other parts, not so much.

As long as you know what you are up against, you're going to emerge victorious and achieve the health benefits you have been yearning for.

At first, you will feel empowered.

Quitting anything will at first give you feelings of power. You are strong enough to quit this, and it wasn't too hard, was it? There are so many recipes you have to choose from, so what's the issue?

Why didn't you do this years ago?

And here come the cravings.

Sugar cravings can creep in starting the next day – or they can take up to ten days to start creeping in. My point is, they *will* come. Some people have reported feeling flu like symptoms, others have reported that they have had actual dreams about bingeing out on sugary sweets.

Though the cravings will come on, and they will be strong, you are stronger than any craving, and you can make it through.

Headaches have also been known to arise.

If you have ever tried to give up caffeine, you know what the headaches feel like. That pounding sensation at your temples – the hollow pounding throughout, it's no fun.

But, just as with caffeine, you will find that sticking with it is your best bet to eliminate it altogether. Within days, your headaches are going to subside, and you will feel better.

The aches and pains of withdrawal.

Though too much sugar intake has been linked to joint and muscle pain, cutting out sugar will have the same effect – at first. As I have already said, some have reported feeling as though they have the flu for up to a week.

However, you don't have to sit back and suffer – nor do you have to give into your cravings. If you are feeling the aches and pains of cutting sugar out of your day, simply take a warm bath with Epsom salts.

Your mood swings may become worse – for a time.

You think you have bad mood swings now, just give yourself some time without sugar. Irritable behavior is one of the most common feelings you will experience when you give up sugar. However, as with the headaches, aches and pains, and other side effects, you are going to only feel the great extent of this for a brief period of time.

Within a week, you'll not only be feeling less irritable, but you will be feeling less anxious and less depressed as well.

You may experience a shaky feeling as you deal with your blood sugar levels adjusting to a life without added sugar.

These may be moderate to severe, and they can be combated by eating something or drinking something without added sugar. This will help alleviate the feelings you are experiencing, and help you get off your sugar addiction.

Then, one day, you are going to wake up feeling better than ever.

Just as you don't know if the adverse effects are going to hit within the first few days or the first week, you don't know if the adverse side effects are going to last for a few days or a few weeks.

But, rest assured, the longer you stick with your new way of life, the easier it's going to be. Sure, it's going to be harder before it gets easier, but with time the cravings and irritability will fade, and you will suddenly see what everyone else who quit sugar is talking about.

You will feel lighter, brighter, and have more energy. You will sleep better at night, and perhaps best of all, you will begin to slim down. Your stomach, love handles, and any other trouble spots on your body will disappear, as well as your skin clearing up.

The biggest thing you must remember as you work through this time is that sugar is addicting. As much as tobacco, nicotine, and some studies even suggest – cocaine. You can't expect to come off an addiction like this without experiencing something.

But it's all worth it. The aches, shakes, and pains, although they seem to take over your day right now, are just bumps along the path to the road of success. Nothing is more empowering than when you have finally rid yourself of this addiction, and start living the life you deserve.

Now, let's get down to the recipes themselves, and put you on the path to the life of success.

Chapter 5 – Sugar Addiction:
How to Beat the Cravings

The throes of withdrawal certainly don't sound like anything pleasant to go through, and I can assure you they aren't going to last forever. However, the longer you keep giving into your sugar cravings, the longer they are going to last.

To beat your addiction and begin your sugar free lifestyle, you must first learn how to get rid of the cravings for good.

Thankfully, there are concrete things you can do that will help you get rid of your sugar cravings. And, with time, beat them altogether. Next time you are having a tough craving, try doing one or two of these things, and watch the craving run its course.

- **Give yourself a treat** – just because you aren't eating sugar it doesn't mean that you can't treat yourself. Try dipping a piece of fruit into some unsweetened chocolate, or eating fruit with a handful of unsweetened chocolate chips.

  Not only are you going to enjoy the sweetness from the fruit, but you will feel satisfied from the indulgence of the chocolate as well.

- **Try chewing on a stick of sugar free** gum – many people who are trying to break their addiction to something turn to gum. It's sweet, it will make you feel as though you are having a real treat, and it's easily available.

  Try fruity or candy flavors (as long as the gum is sugar free) and you'll be kicking that craving in no time.

- **Walk away** – next time a tough sugar craving hits, try walking around the block or getting up and doing some jumping jacks. The rush of exercise will send a flood of endorphins from your brain, making you feel happy and satisfied – all without the sugar.

  Plus, if you aren't in the same room as the sugary treats, you will be less tempted to try them.

- **Eat regularly** – this is especially important when you are in the initial stages of quitting sugar. It is easy to associate sugar with hunger, largely because your body is low on blood sugar when you are hungry.

  If you are careful to eat regularly, you will be less hungry throughout the day, you decrease your chances of experiencing a tough craving.

- **If you have to, and *only* if you have to, allow yourself to indulge (a little.)** – everyone is different, and to be perfectly honest, quitting cold turkey just isn't feasible for some people. If you simply must have something sweet (meaning candy or some kind of similar treat) allow yourself to indulge, as long as you keep it in perspective. If you totally deprive yourself, even during the worst symptoms, it could backfire and you may end up bingeing later.

  Instead of total deprivation, opt for quality of your treat over quantity of your treat. If you are going to eat a piece of candy, you are much better of savoring a single rich chocolate truffle than you are a somewhat sweet candy bar.

  Indulge in each little nibble you take, and enjoy the treat, then move on and forget about it.

Once you realize that sugar is an addiction, you will be better able to break free of it by using the right strategies. Don't beat yourself up over how you are feeling, and if you do choose to indulge a little, do it and move on.

The more you work on getting rid of the addiction, the less the cravings will come, and the less severe they will be when they do occur. At the end of the day, strategy is going to get you off of sugar and help you live your zero sugar lifestyle for the long haul.

Trust me, you will feel better, and with time, the sugar isn't going to taste nearly as good as it does right now. Give yourself time, and in the end, you will triumph.

Remember by going sugar free you are not using foods with added sugar. This doesn't include the naturally occurring sugars in foods such as fruits or milk.

For allergies, substitutes have been provided.

Sugar Free Sweet Waffles

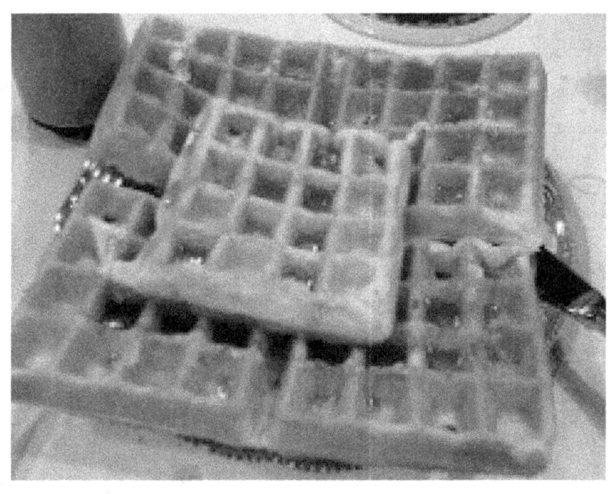

Serves 6 Sugar og

What you will need:

2 cups whole wheat flour

½ teaspoon baking soda

1 teaspoon baking powder

1 teaspoon salt

2 teaspoons cinnamon

1 tablespoon powdered stevia

3 eggs, beaten

2 ounces unsalted butter

1 teaspoon vanilla

2 cups buttermilk

Directions:

Soften the butter and combine all the dry ingredients. Beat the eggs then stir them into the mix, then add the vanilla, buttermilk. Mix until it is a batter consistency.

Heat your waffle iron according to the directions, then scoop the batter onto the waffle iron. This recipe will make 6 waffles.

Substitutions:

Egg – use ¼ cup unsweetened applesauce per egg

Dairy – use a nut milk or hemp milk. Make sure you opt for unsweetened milk regardless of which you choose.

Flour - use a nut flour or coconut flour

Ever Delicious Oatmeal Muffins

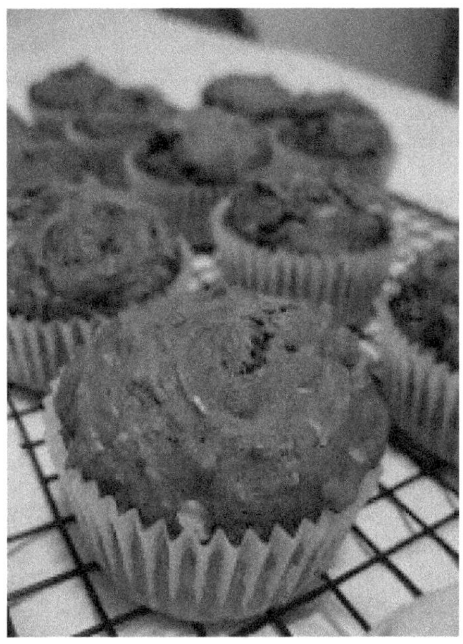

Serves 12 Sugar 1.4g

What you will need:

1 cup rolled oats

½ cup ground flaxseed

1 teaspoon baking powder

1 teaspoon cinnamon

½ teaspoon salt

2 eggs

1 teaspoon vanilla extract

½ teaspoon liquid vanilla stevia

½ cup milk

2 smashed bananas (this will be about 1 cup)

Directions:

Preheat your oven to 350 degrees F.

In a large bowl, use your hand mixer to combine the dry ingredients first, then add in the wet ingredients next. Continue to mix until smooth.

Line a muffin tin with muffin liners, or spray them with no stick cooking spray. There will be enough batter to make a total of 12 muffins.

Pour the batter into the muffin tins, then place in the oven and bake for 20 minutes.

Transfer to a wire rack to cool, then enjoy.

Egg – use ¼ cup unsweetened applesauce per egg

Dairy – use a nut milk or hemp milk. Make sure you opt for unsweetened milk regardless of which you choose.

Heavenly Oatmeal (Slow Cooker Version)

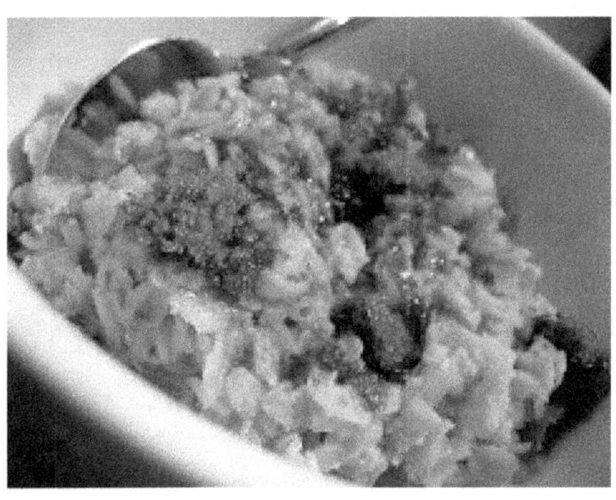

Serves 4 Sugar 0g

What you will need:
2 cups milk
1 cup rolled oats
1 tablespoon butter
½ teaspoon cinnamon
1 tablespoon liquid stevia
¼ teaspoon salt

Directions:

Combine all ingredients in your favorite slow cooker, and turn onto low. Cook overnight, or for about 8 hours.

Stir well, and serve with your toppings of choice.

Substitutions:

Dairy free – leave out the butter and use nut or hemp milk of choice. Make sure you opt for unsweetened milk regardless of which you choose.

Busy Morning Sugar Free Oatmeal

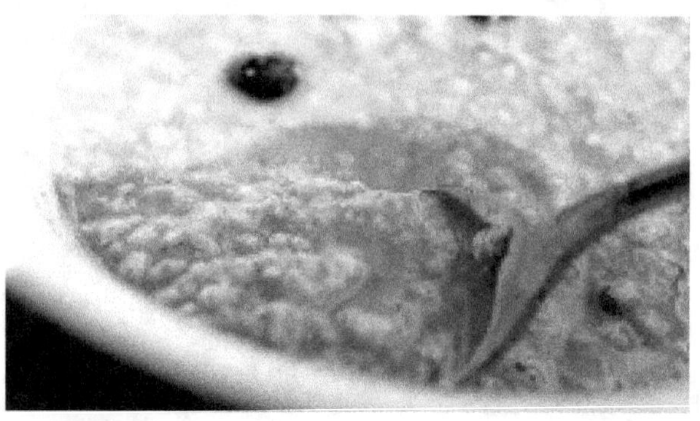

Serves 4 Sugar 0g

What you will need:

2 cups milk

1 cup rolled oats

1 tablespoon liquid stevia

¼ teaspoon salt

1 teaspoon nutmeg

Directions:

Heat the milk over medium heat in a medium saucepan on the stove. Once the milk is hot, pour in the rest of the ingredients, stir, and cover.

Allow to cook for 5 minutes, then uncover.

Stir well, and serve with your toppings of choice.

Substitutions:

Dairy free – leave out the butter and use nut or hemp milk of choice. Make sure you opt for unsweetened milk regardless of which you choose.

Soaked Fruity Oats

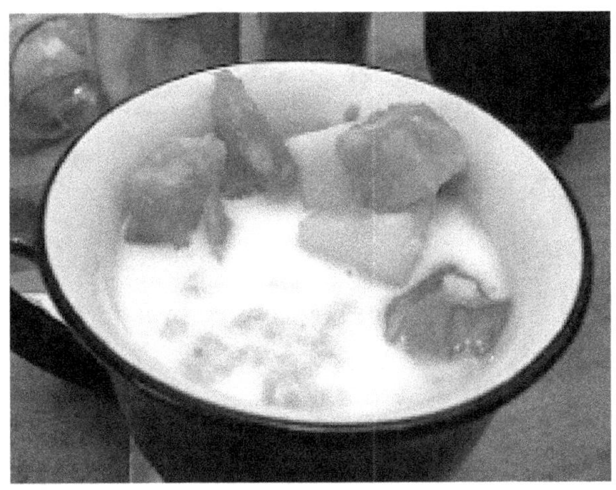

Serves 1 Sugars 0g

What you will need:

¼ cup rolled oats

1 tablespoon chia seeds

1/3 cup almond milk

¼ cup plain Greek yogurt

½ teaspoon stevia, vanilla flavored

½ teaspoon vanilla extract

1 chopped champagne mango, chopped into bite sized pieces

Directions:

Be careful as you chop the mango, they are slippery and can easily cause injury. Transfer all ingredients into a pint sized jar, and cover in the fridge overnight or for 8 hours.

In the morning, give the ingredients a stir and enjoy.

Substitutions:

Yogurt – use a nut yogurt or soy yogurt for a dairy free version of this recipe

Almond milk – use hemp milk if you are allergic to nuts, or use regular milk if you do not want a dairy free version of the recipe. Make sure you opt for unsweetened milk regardless of which you choose.

Chocolate Chia Sugar Free Delight

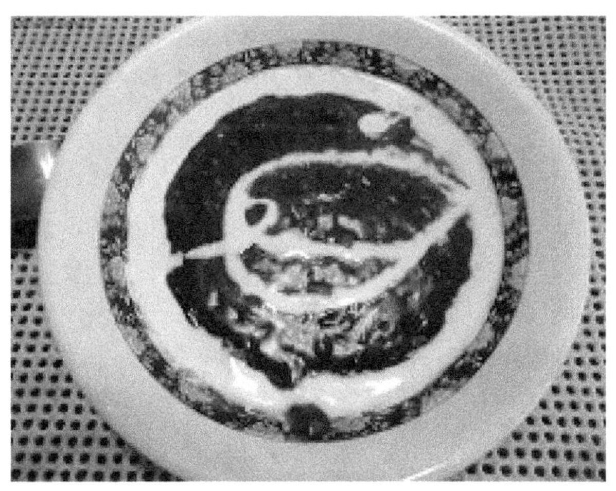

Serves 1 Sugar 0g

What you will need:

¼ cup rolled oats

¼ cup Greek yogurt

1/3 cup almond milk

1 tablespoon chia seeds

½ tablespoon sugar free peanut butter

2 teaspoons stevia – chocolate flavored

Directions:

Combine all ingredients in a bowl and stir well. Transfer all the ingredients to a suitably sized jar and leave in the fridge overnight, or for at least 8 hours.

Stir well, and enjoy.

Substitutions:

Yogurt – use a nut yogurt or soy yogurt for a dairy free version of this recipe. Make sure you opt for unsweetened product regardless of which you choose.

Almond milk – use hemp milk if you are allergic to nuts, or use regular milk if you do not want a dairy free version of the recipe

Delectable French Toast Bites

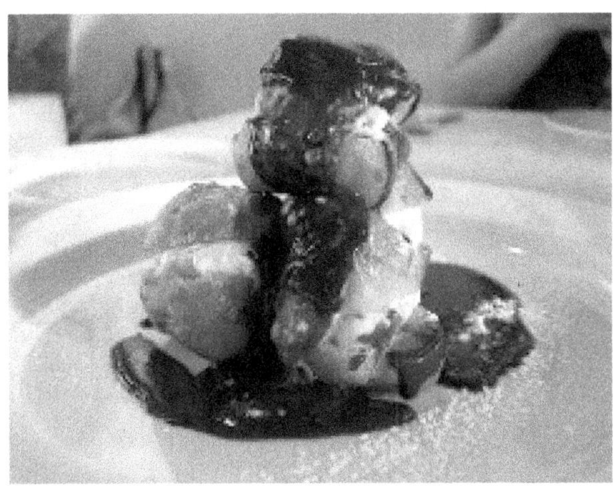

Serves 8 Sugars 11g

What you will need:

6 eggs

½ cup egg whites

1 can light coconut milk

2 teaspoons ground cinnamon

2 teaspoons liquid stevia

2 teaspoons vanilla extract

2 tablespoons ground extract

5 cups gluten free bread of choice

For the cinnamon crumble:

1 cup quick oats

1 cup shredded unsweetened coconut

2 teaspoons ground cinnamon

1 teaspoon salt

1 teaspoon ground cloves

2 teaspoons vanilla extract

¼ cup honey

¼ cup coconut oil, melted or fractionated

Directions:

Preheat your oven to 350 degrees F.

Combine the first 7 ingredients on the list, everything except for the bread crumbles and set aside. In another dish, combine the remaining ingredients except for the bread once again.

Tear the bread into bite sized pieces.

Grease a baking dish, then add the bread to this dish. Add the egg mixture to the brad first, then the cinnamon mixture to the dish next. Place in the oven and bake for 50 minutes, until the center of the mix looks firm.

Serve with the topping of your choice.

Substitutions:

Egg – Use ¼ cup unsweetened applesauce per egg

Honey – Use 3 tablespoons of stevia in place of the honey to lower the sugar content to nearly 0g

Remember by going sugar free you are not using foods with added sugar. This doesn't include the naturally occurring sugars in foods such as fruits or milk.

For allergies, substitutes have been provided.

Beef 'n' Peppers

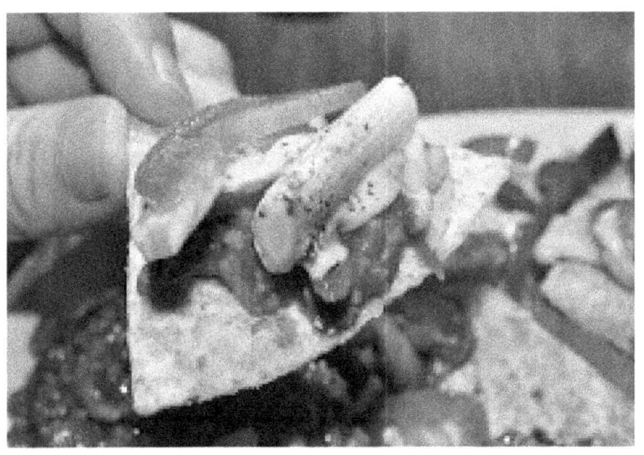

Serves 2 Sugars 0g

What you will need:

½ pound ground beef

1 onion

1 cup spinach

Salt

Pepper

1 bell pepper

Directions:

Brown the burger over medium heat in a pan on the stove, and season with salt and pepper to taste. Slice the onion into leaves, and slice the bell pepper. Remove the seeds from the bell pepper, then add the onion and bell pepper to the burger.

Add the spinach last, and allow to cook for another 5 minutes, until the spinach has just begun to wilt.

Serve immediately, with chips, if desired.

Forky Cheeseburgers

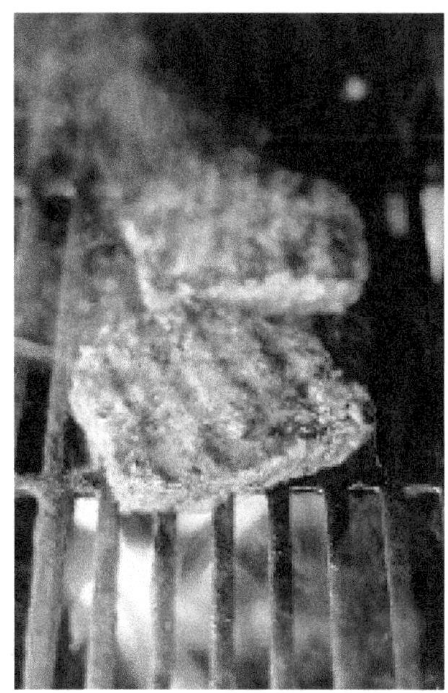

Serves 2 Sugars 1.2g

What you will need:

1 pound ground burger

2 slices cheddar cheese

½ brick cream cheese

Salt

Pepper

Sugar free salsa

1 cup spinach

Directions:

Form the burger into 2 patties with your hands, and heat a pan over medium heat on the stove. Transfer the burgers to the heated pan, and wash your hands thoroughly.

Soften the cream cheese in the microwave, then mix with the cheddar cheese. Season the burger with salt and pepper to taste.

When the burgers are done cooking, add the cheese to each one and allow to melt slightly.

Transfer to 2 plates, and top with the spinach and the salsa. Serve immediately.

Substitutions:

Dairy free – use vegan Daiya cheddar cheese substitute for the cheddar, use tofu for the cream cheese.

Curried Chicken Bites

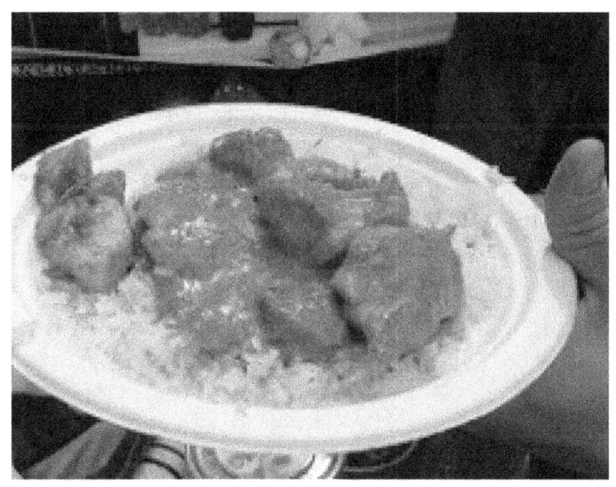

Serves 2 Sugar 0g

What you will need:

2 boneless skinless chicken breasts

1 tablespoon butter

Salt

Pepper

2 teaspoons curry powder

2 carrot sticks

1 celery stick

Directions:

Heat a pan over medium heat on the stove, and cut the chicken into bite sized pieces. Allow the butter to melt in the pan, then add the chicken in next. As the chicken is cooking, wash the veggies and coin them.

Add these to the chicken when it has been cooked thoroughly, and season with the salt, pepper, and curry powder.

Cover, and allow to simmer on the stove for 5 minutes. Serve immediately.

Substitutions:

Dairy free – Use 1 tablespoon coconut oil instead of the butter

Delectable Tuna Salad

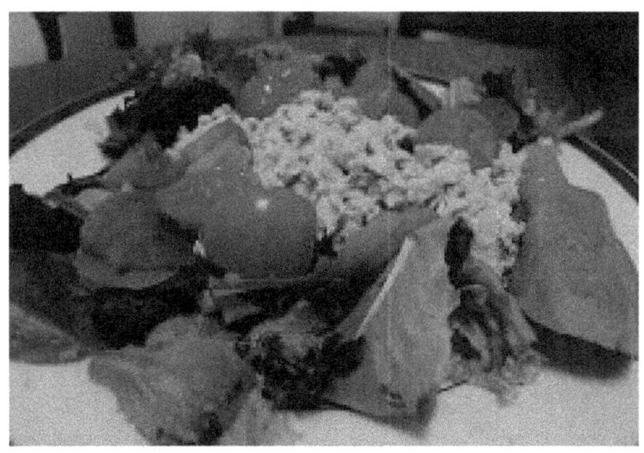

Serves 1 Sugars 3g

What you will need:

1 cup romaine lettuce

½ red onion, sliced

1 small can black olives

½ cup Roma tomatoes, sliced in half

2 hard boiled eggs, sliced

1 can tuna, opened and drained

For the dressing:

¼ cup olive oil

¼ cup white vinegar

1 teaspoon honey

1 teaspoon snipped tarragon

1 teaspoon dried brown mustard

¼ teaspoon salt

Black pepper

Directions:

Prepare the veggies, eggs, and tuna as directed in the ingredient list. Pile in a large bowl.

For the dressing, combine the ingredients for the dressing, mixing quickly so they blend well. Top the salad with the dressing, then toss to coat.

Serve immediately.

Substitutions:

Eggs – the eggs can be substituted for ½ cup tuna

Tuna – the tuna can be substituted for ½ cup shredded chicken, or left off altogether

Honey – the honey can be substituted for 2 teaspoons stevia, bringing the sugar content down to 0g

Home Made Mac 'n' Cheese

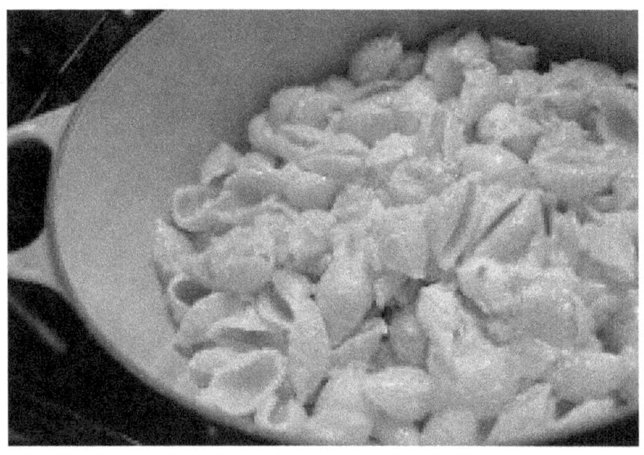

Serves 2 Sugar 0g

What you will need:

2 cups pasta

1 tablespoon butter

1 cup shredded cheddar cheese

1 tablespoon mustard

½ cup white flour

¾ cup milk

Salt

Pepper

Directions:

Boil the pasta according to the packaging directions. Pour into a colander to drain.

In your pan, add the milk, butter, and cheese, and continue to stir until it has melted. Add the remaining ingredients, stirring until a smooth sauce. Add the macaroni back into the mix, and stir.

Serve immediately.

Substitutions:

Pasta – use a gluten free pasta or cauliflower

Cheddar cheese – use the vegan Daiya cheddar cheese

Milk – use nut or hemp milk. Make sure you opt for unsweetened milk regardless of which you choose.

Butter – use 1 tablespoon coconut oil

Creamy Tomato Soup

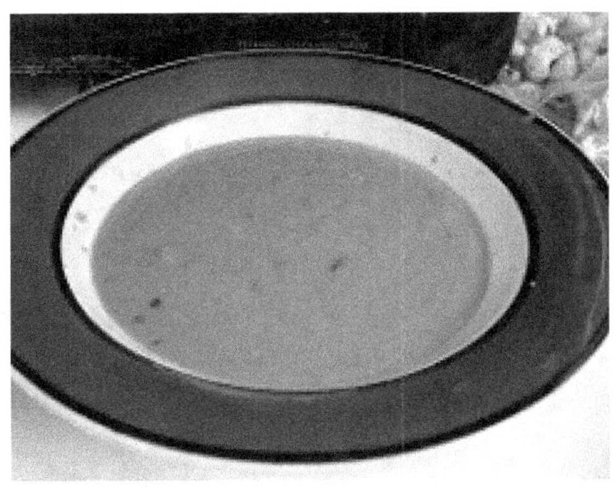

Serves 2 Sugars 0g

What you will need:

1 can tomato sauce

2 cups milk

Salt

Pepper

Basil

1 can sugar free diced tomatoes

Directions:

Open and drain the can of diced tomatoes, then combine all ingredients in a saucepan on the stove.

Heat thoroughly until heated through, and serve.

Substitutions:

Dairy free version – use nut milk or hemp milk of your choice. Make sure you opt for unsweetened milk regardless of which you choose.

Chicken Strips

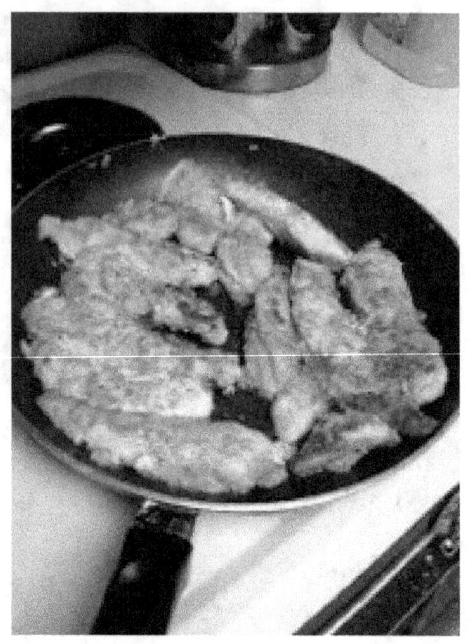

Serves 1 Sugars 0g

What you will need:

1 boneless skinless chicken breast

1 egg

3 tablespoons milk

¼ cup flour

Salt

Pepper

Directions:

Preheat oven to 350 degrees F.

Slice the chicken into strips, and whisk the milk and the egg together in a bowl. In a separate bowl, combine 1 teaspoon of salt with 1 teaspoon of pepper and the flour.

Take your strips of chicken and dip them first in the egg wash, then roll them in the flour mix, coating evenly. Gently knock the chicken against the sides of the bowl to remove any of the excess breading, then place on a greased baking sheet.

Bake in the oven 30 to 40 minutes, flipping the strips over halfway through. They are done when the breading is a golden brown and the chicken is cooked through.

Serve with your favorite sugar free dipping sauce.

Substitutions:

Flour – for a low carb or gluten free version use nut or coconut flour of your choice

Milk – use either a nut milk, hemp milk, or soy milk of your choice. Make sure you opt for unsweetened milk regardless of which you choose.

Egg – leave this out and add another tablespoon of milk

Remember by going sugar free you are not using foods with added sugar. This doesn't include the naturally occurring sugars in foods such as fruits or milk.

For allergies, substitutes have been provided.

Best Ever Gnocchi

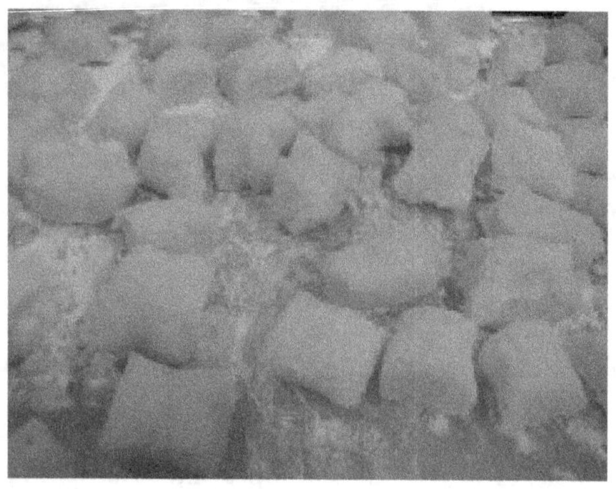

Serves 6 Sugar 0g

What you will need:

3 cups cauliflower

1 cup grated parmesan

2 egg yolks

1 tsp garlic powder

½ tsp salt

¼ tsp pepper

1 tsp xanthan gum

¾ cup coconut flour

12 ounce mozzarella cheese

Directions:

Start by cooking the cauliflower thoroughly, then mashing it with either a hand masher, your food processer, or a food mixer.

Transfer to a large bowl (or continue to use your food processor, if this is what you are using) and add in the rest of the ingredients, except for the mozzarella cheese.

Melt the mozzarella in either the microwave or on the stove. Be careful and watch it as you melt it so it does not burn. This will take roughly 1 or 2 minutes in the microwave, or constant supervision and stirring on the stove.

After you have melted the mozzarella, transfer it into the bowl with the rest of the batter and mix well.

Once the dough has been formed, roll into gnocchi shapes and use a fork to leave the marks on the top. Line a pan with parchment paper, then place all of these onto the parchment paper and place in the freezer for at least 1 hour.

When you are ready to use, boil a large pot of water, then transfer the gnocchi into the water. Boil for 2 minutes, then transfer to another pan to saute with your favorite sugar free sauce.

Simmer on the stove for 5 minutes, then serve with parmesan cheese.

Substitutions:

2 egg yolks – use ¼ cup apple sauce (unsweetened) in place of the egg yolks.

Parmesan cheese – use a vegan parmesan cheese substitute for the same flavor and texture.

Mozzarella cheese – use the vegan Daiya mozzarella cheese instead of dairy mozzarella cheese.

Flour – use any nut flour of choice, or use wheat flour if that is what you would prefer.

Cheesy Zucchini Cups

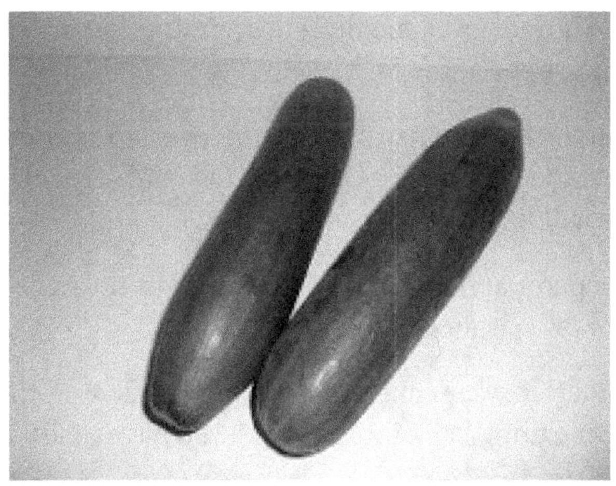

Serves 6 Sugars 2g

What you will need:

3 zucchini

8 ounces burger

3 ounces chopped onion

4 ounces cream cheese

3 ounces fresh spinach

Directions:

Brown the burger over medium heat on the stove with a dash of salt and pepper, if desired.

As the burger is cooking, preheat the oven to 350 degrees F. and wash the Zucchini. Cut the zucchini the short way, creating small logs rather than long boats.

Use your spoon and scoop out the center of the zucchini, and add this to the burger on the stove.

Finally, add the cream cheese to the burger as well, then begin scooping this filing back into the cups you have made.

Line a baking sheet with foil, and place each of the stuffed cups on the baking sheet.

Place in the oven and bake for 30 minutes, then serve hot.

Substitutions:

Dairy free version – use tofu in place of the cream cheese for the same texture.

Everyone's Favorite Spaghetti

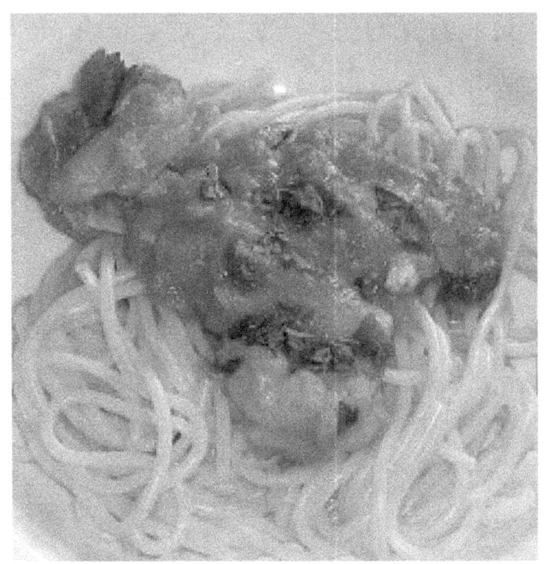

Serves 4 Sugars 1g

What you will need:

1 package spaghetti

1 pound burger

Salt

Pepper

1 teaspoon basil

1 jar sugar free tomato sauce

1 onion

1 jar olives

1 teaspoon garlic powder

Directions:

Prepare the pasta according to the packaging directions.

While the pasta is cooking, brown the burger over medium heat on the stove, chop the onion, and open and drain the can of olives. Chop the olives as small as you can get them, then transfer the onions and the olives to the hamburger.

Season with all the seasonings, then add the tomato sauce. If the sauce is too thick, add in a can of water as well.

Allow the meat to simmer for 10 minutes, and once the pasta has finished cooking, serve the sauce over the pasta.

Substitutions:

Gluten free version – use a gluten free pasta, or substitute spaghetti squash for the wheat pasta instead.

World's Best Shepherd's Pie

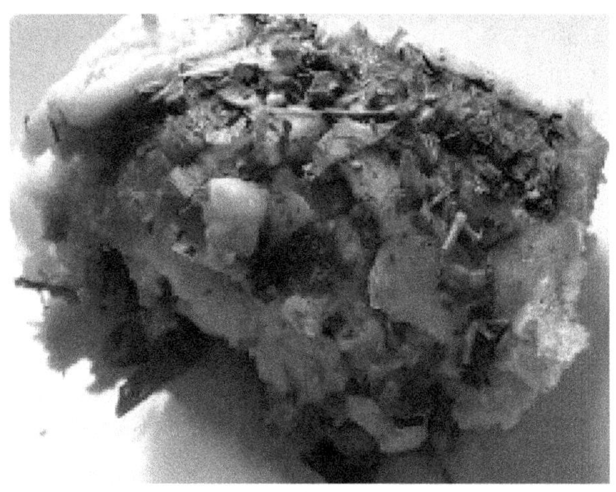

Serves 4 Sugar 1g

What you will need:

2 cups mashed potatoes

Salt

Pepper

Paprika

1 pound burger

1 onion

2 cans green beans

Directions:

Chop the onion and put it in the pan to brown with the burger over medium heat on the stove. Continue to cook until the burger has been cooked through, and until the onion has become translucent.

Preheat the oven to 350 degrees F. and spray a baking pan with no stick cooking spray. Transfer the meat mixture to the baking dish and set aside.

Open and drain the cans of green beans, then place these in next over the meat mix, spreading them out so the meat is covered.

Season with salt and pepper, then spread the mashed potatoes over the top like frosting.

Garnish next with the paprika, adding a pleasant color to the top. Cover the dish with foil, and place in the oven to bake for 20 minutes.

Serve immediately.

Sweet Potato Delight

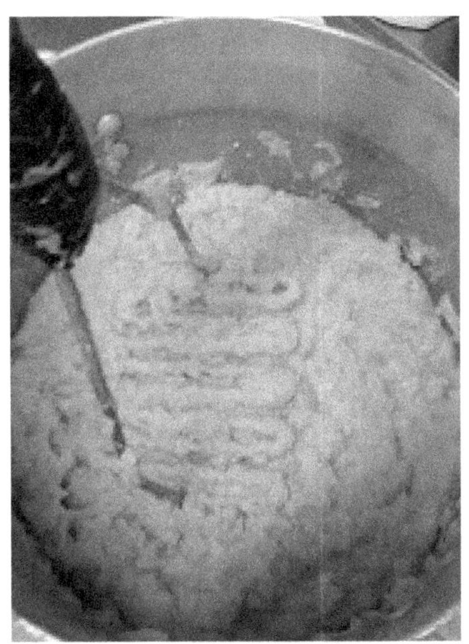

Serves 2 Sugars 0g

What you will need:

3 sweet potatoes

1 butternut squash

½ teaspoon ground cinnamon

½ teaspoon nutmeg

¼ cup sugar free maple flavored syrup

Directions:

Peel both the sweet potatoes and the squash. Cut the sweet potatoes into cubes and boil them for 10 minutes on the stove, until they are soft. Smash the sweet potatoes with the squash, then mix in the seasonings.

Heat another pan on the stove, and lightly spray with no stick cooking spray. Form the sweet potato mix into patties. There will be enough to make 6 patties.

Cook the sweet potato mix on the stove, about 3 to 4 minutes per side, until cooked.

Transfer back to the plates, and serve with a garnishing of syrup.

Enjoy immediately.

Baked Peppers

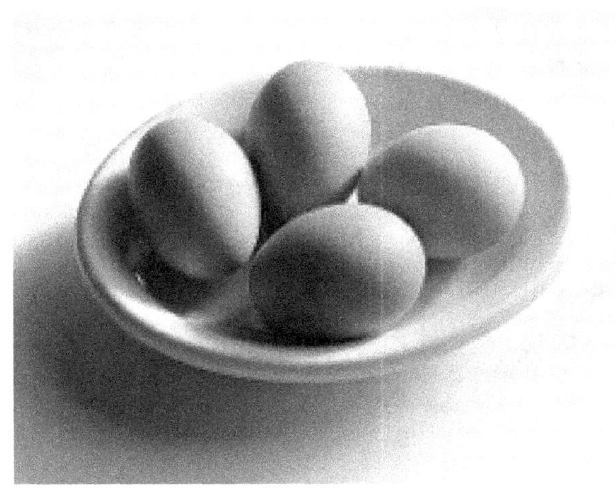

Serves 1 Sugars 0g

What you will need:

2 eggs

1 red pepper

Salt

Pepper

1 teaspoon parsley

Directions:

Preheat the oven to 350 degrees F. and spray a baking sheet with no stick cooking spray.

Slice the peppers in half the short way rather than in half – opposite of what you normally would. Scoop out the centers of these peppers, and wash thoroughly.

Crack an egg into each of these pepper halves, and season with salt and pepper to taste. Garnish with the parsley, then place in the oven to bake.

Bake for 20 to 30 minutes, until the eggs are cooked through.

Serve immediately.

Substitutions:

Egg free version – cut an avocado in half and smash with ¼ cup parmesan cheese. Stuff the pepper with this mix, and bake as you normally would.

Egg free and dairy free version – use the avocado as you normally would, but instead of using parmesan cheese, use a vegan variation of parmesan – it's dairy free and has the same taste.

Stuff the pepper with this and bake as you normally would.

Zucchini Pizza Bites

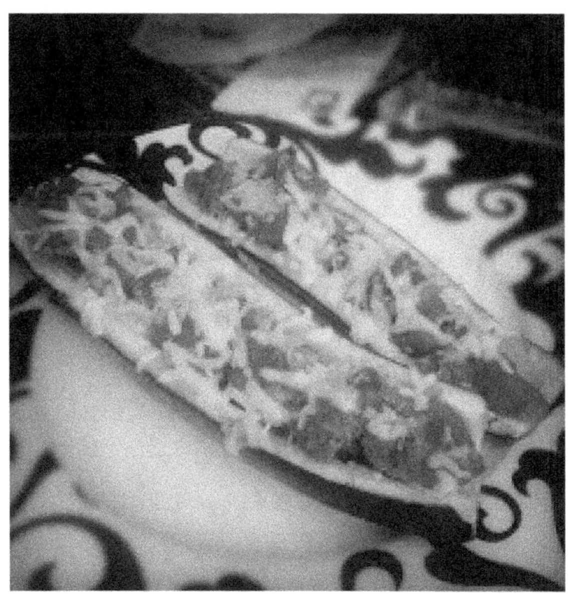

Serves 2 Sugar 1g

What you will need:

2 zucchini

1 jar sugar free tomato sauce

½ pound hamburger

1 package mozzarella

2 teaspoons basil

1 teaspoon garlic powder

1 jar olives, opened, drained, and chopped

Salt

Pepper

Directions:

Wash the zucchini and cut them into 1 inch thick coins. Line a baking sheet with foil, and place the zucchini on the baking sheet.

Preheat your oven to 350 degrees F. and brown the burger in a pan over medium heat on the stove.

Open the jar of tomato sauce, and mix the sauce with the seasonings. Layer the ingredients on the zucchini as you would a pizza – first the sauce, then the cheese, then the burger and olives.

Place the pan in the oven and bake for 30 to 40 minutes, until cooked through and the cheese is melted. Serve immediately.

Substitutions:

Dairy free version – instead of using mozzarella cheese, use the Daiya mozzarella style cheese shreds, they taste virtually the same and have the same texture, but they are vegan and completely dairy free.

Remember by going sugar free you are not using foods with added sugar. This doesn't include the naturally occurring sugars in foods such as fruits or milk.

For allergies, substitutes have been provided.

Chocolate Chia Pudding

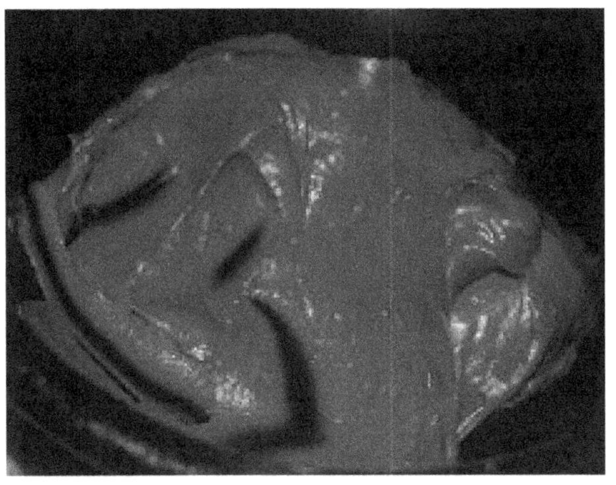

Serves 1 Sugar 0g

What you will need:

1 cup milk

1 tablespoon stevia extract, chocolate flavored

2 tablespoons chia seeds

1 teaspoon vanilla

Directions:

Combine all ingredients in a bowl and mix well. Place plastic wrap over the top of the bowl, allowing it to droop down and touch the top of the pudding mix.

Place in the fridge and allow to sit from 8 hours to overnight.

Remove the plastic wrap from the pudding, stir, and serve.

Substitutions:

Dairy free version – use nut milk or hemp milk of your choice, just make sure you use the unsweetened version of any milk you choose.

Quick 'n' Easy Ice Cream

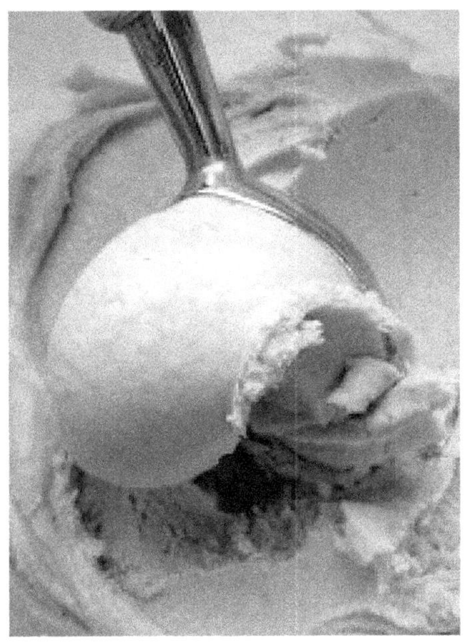

Serves 1 Sugar 0g

What you will need:

2 bananas

2 packets stevia extract

1 tablespoon vanilla

Directions:

Cut the bananas into coins and place in the freezer. Leave them in the freezer for at least 4 hours.

Transfer frozen bananas to your blender, and add the vanilla and stevia.

Blend lightly until the bananas have the texture of ice cream.

Serve and enjoy immediately.

Dipped Indulgence

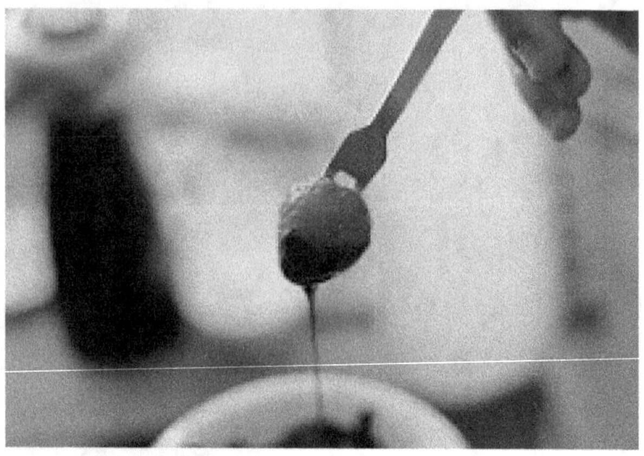

Serves 2 Sugars 2g

What you will need:

2 cups strawberries

2 cups unsweetened chocolate chips

2 tablespoons stevia extract, chocolate flavored

2 tablespoons almond milk, unsweetened

Directions:

In a saucepan on the stove, combine the chocolate chips, stevia, and almond milk. Turn on to low, and keep an eye on it as you stir occasionally, making sure it doesn't burn.

Continue to stir until the chocolate is completely melted. Wash the strawberries, then use a fork to dip them into the chocolate.

Enjoy immediately, or allow to harden with the chocolate on top.

Substitutions:

Dairy version – use regular milk in place of the almond milk.

Dairy free version – use vegan chocolate chips in place of the normal chocolate chips.

Nut free version – use regular milk or unsweetened hemp milk in place of the almond milk.

Insanely Fudge

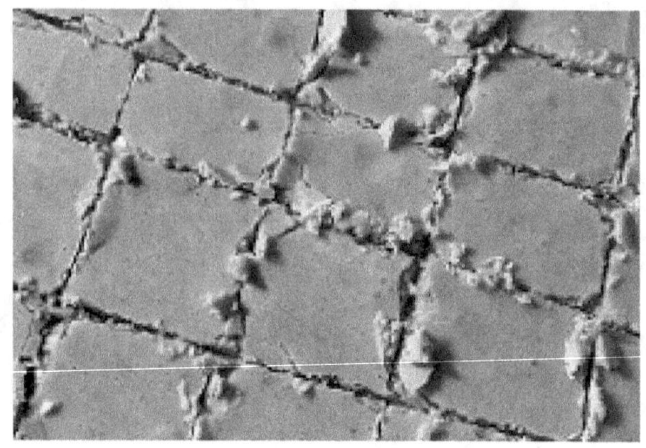

Serves 16 Sugars 0.6g

What you will need:

4 ounces raw, unsalted sunflower seeds

4 ounces sunbutter

2 scoops chocolate protein powder

3 ounces unsweetened cocoa powder

4 tablespoons stevia

½ tsp salt

8 tablespoons coconut oil

Directions:

Using either a food processor or a blender, combine all ingredients and blend on medium. Continue to blend until all ingredients have mixed or climbed up on the sides, then take a spatula and scrape them back down, before blending again.

Line a pan with parchment paper while the blender is running, and once you have completely blended the ingredients, transfer them to the pan with the parchment paper.

Place in the fridge for half an hour. Slice into 16 bars.

Store in the fridge and enjoy whenever you are ready.

Heavenly Parfait

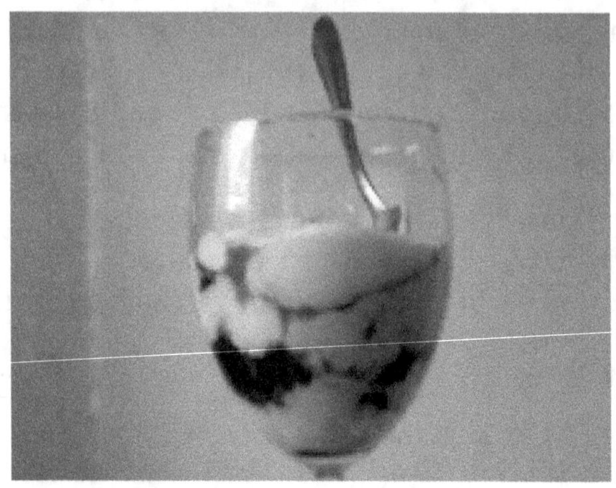

Serves 1 Sugar 0g

What you will need:

1 cup plain Greek yogurt

1 teaspoon vanilla

½ cup raspberries

½ cup almonds

Directions:

Gently combine the vanilla with the yogurt, being careful not to ruin the composition of the yogurt in the process.

Place 1 scoop of yogurt at the bottom of a tall flute, then the raspberries. Follow with more yogurt, then add the nuts. Finish with the rest of the yogurt, and serve immediately.

Substitutions:

Dairy free version – instead of using Greek yogurt, try a nut or soy yogurt instead, just make sure you stick with buying only the unsweetened varieties of whatever you choose.

Nut free version – instead of using a layer of nuts, try adding in another layer of raspberries, or another kind of berry such as strawberries or blueberries.

Chocolate Crunch Bites

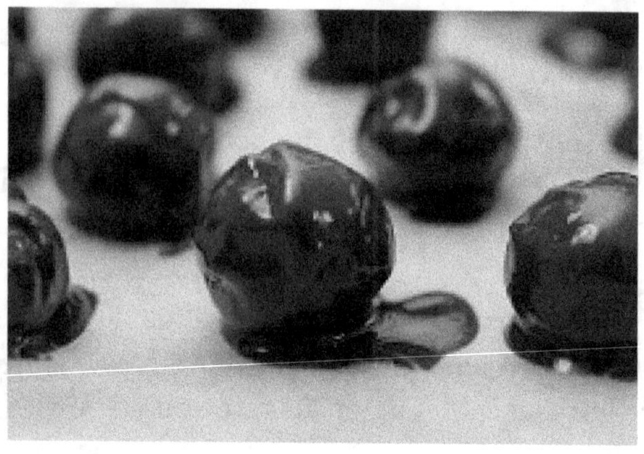

Serves 6 Sugar 0g

What you will need:

¾ cup shredded unsweetened coconut

¼ cup unsweetened cocoa powder

¼ cup hemp hearts

¼ raw, unsalted pumpkin seeds

¼ raw, unsalted sunflower seeds

½ cup sunflower seed butter

¼ teaspoon salt

½ teaspoon stevia extract

½ teaspoon chocolate stevia extract

Directions:

In a large bowl with a hand mixer, or with your food processor, combine all the ingredients and blend until they are as smooth as you can get them.

If you are using a food processor (or something similar, such as a blender) you will need to scrape the batter down from the sides of the bowl as it climbs to the top.

After the batter has been blended until smooth, line a sheet with parchment paper, then grab small handfuls of the dough and roll them into balls between your palms.

There will be enough to make 6 balls.

Store in the fridge for at least 4 hours, up to overnight before serving.

Substitutes:

If you are unable to eat coconut – use chopped dates or chopped plums instead. They will change the texture of the balls slightly, but they might even make them taste more chocolatey than before.

To Die For Strawberry Cheesecake

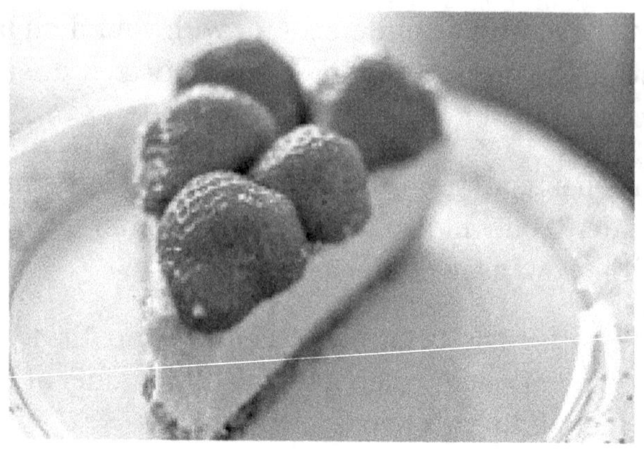

Serves 6 Sugar 0g

What you will need:

¾ cup graham cracker crumbs

2 tablespoons butter, melted

¼ teaspoon ground cinnamon

¼ teaspoon ground nutmeg

1 package cream cheese, softened

1 ½ cups milk

1 package cheesecake flavor sugar free instant pudding mix

2 pints fresh strawberries, sliced

Directions:

Combine all the seasonings with the graham cracker crumbs in a bowl, then add the melted butter to the mix. Press this mix into the bottom of an 8 inch pie pan, making sure you spread the crust all the way to the edges, then storing in the fridge while you mix the rest of the ingredients.

Soften the cream cheese by mixing it with a hand mixer in a large bowl. Once softened, add the pudding mix and the milk. Continue to mix until smooth.

Once you have this batter well mixed, gently pour into the crust you have waiting in the fridge. Allow to sit in the fridge for 4 hours, until the cake begins to set up.

Lay the strawberries on top of the cheesecake, carefully placing them so they do not ruin the cake that has not fully set up. Return to the fridge for another 2 to 4 hours, until completely firm.

Slice and serve when you are ready.

Substitutions:

Dairy free version – use the nut or hemp milk of your choice, just remember to opt for the unsweetened version of any milk you choose for your dessert. For the cream cheese, you can substitute that with GO VEGGIE vegan cream cheese. It has the same texture and flavor as regular cream cheese, but you don't need to use any dairy.

To substitute the butter simply add 2 tablespoons of coconut oil, and you are ready to indulge.

Conclusion

There you have it, everything you need to get started on the zero sugar diet, and what you need to know that will help you stick with it for the long term. I hope this book was able to give you the inspiration you need to start the zero sugar diet for yourself, and to turn it into your lifestyle.

Making a change is hard. We as people are wired to do things as we have always done them. To live life as we have always lived it, and to be who we have always been.

But, this may not be the best for your health, and unless you make some critical changes, you may be headed for some rough seas in your life. From the threat of chronic illness to obesity, struggling with your sleep schedule, and having energy during the day, sugar can affect every part of your life.

However, when you make the decision to change your diet, you may feel overwhelmed. There are so many things filled with sugar, it's nearly impossible to find food that doesn't have any added.

Or is it?

I hope this book was able to show you that if you make foods yourself, you are able to decide exactly what goes into them, and control the amount of sugar you are eating.

There's no end to the way you can cut sugar out of your life, and enjoy a life of natural foods. Yes, this is something that is hard to do at first, but if you are willing to make the change, and you are willing to stick with the changes you have made, you will quickly see the benefits unfold in your life.

Not only will your body change physically, but it will also change mentally, giving you peace and happiness as you have always wanted. Who would have guessed that sugar could take such a toll on your life?

Knowledge is the key to health, and now that you know how to break free of your sugar addiction, you have put yourself on the right track to health and happiness.

So what are you waiting for?

Your sugar free, happy and energetic life awaits, and it is oh, so sweet.

Good luck!

www.ingramcontent.com/pod-product-compliance
Lightning Source LLC
Chambersburg PA
CBHW071233240726

48654CB00009B/1033